# The Well Mom, Well Baby Guide:

## *Simple, Effective Strategies for a Happy Journey Together.*

# Velma W. Price

# TABLE OF CONTENT

# INTRODUCTION

## Setting the Stage for a Healthy Journey Together

Emma watched in a mix of astonishment and disbelief as the late afternoon sun sank below the horizon, casting a warm, golden glow across the small, comfortable hospital room. Her newborn son lay nestled in her arms, his tiny fingers curling and uncurling as if exploring this new world. Emma was awestruck; he had finally arrived. She was now a mother. Looking down at him, emotions swirled within her—joy, love, and a touch of apprehension.

An unbreakable bond surged within her, accompanied by a deep sense of purpose and questions both big and small. Was he warm enough? Should she let him sleep or continue holding him close? With the overwhelming need to love, care for, and protect this tiny life now woven into every breath, she wondered how she'd ever sleep again.

She experienced an unshakable connection and a newfound feeling of purpose. However, that goal came with both big and minor questions. Was he sufficiently warm? Should she let him sleep or hold him? And with the overpowering need to love, care for, and protect this tiny life now woven into every breath, how was she supposed to sleep?

A soft knock at her door broke the stillness of the evening. Maria, her nurse, entered with a kind and compassionate grin. As she pulled up a chair next to the bed she said, "How are you feeling, Emma?" All of the thoughts Emma had attempted to suppress since giving birth flooded her consciousness.

Maria was able to read her thoughts. "You know, when I had my first baby, I thought I'd read everything there was to know," she added with a quiet laugh. I believed that I was ready! But doesn't parenting have a way of taking us by surprise? She extended her hand and gave the infant's cheek a soft, well-practiced pat. "Emma, nobody can know all the answers. However, we gradually discover what suits us and our children the best. Finding simple and enjoyable ways to incorporate them into our lives is crucial.

Attracted by Maria's serene demeanour, Emma raised her head. She could see that Maria had experienced this previously and that she was aware of Emma's joys and concerns. Maria started telling stories about the small things that had aided her in navigating her path, rather than about perfection or quick fixes. "I discovered that even the tiniest rituals and habits had a significant impact. For example, I was taking a moment to myself when I needed it most or learning how to breathe during stressful situations. I understood that if I were well, my child would also be well.

Emma felt a wave of relief begin to wash over her as Maria talked. There was a feeling of acceptance and a reassuring reminder that parenthood wasn't about making everything perfect right away. Finding balance was key, involving easy routines, doable tactics, and small acts of self-compassion so she could give her all to her child.

Maria came back the following morning with a notebook. She gave it to Emma and said, "This is for you." Inside, she had jotted down some of the tactics and advice that had aided her over the years, things she believed would provide direction and solace for Emma's path. Maria clarified, "We can't predict everything, but we can find little ways to make each day a little brighter, a little easier." "We can provide even better care for our children when we take care of ourselves. It's about creating a long-lasting foundation for wellness.

As Emma turned the pages, she felt the weight of this straightforward manual in her hands, like a tiny road map that would guide her through the somewhat confusing world of new parenthood. There were reminders to be patient and kind to herself, suggestions for basic self-care, and advice on routines for both mother and child. Even sections devoted to typical obstacles and their elegant and straightforward solutions were included.

Maria smiled and remarked, "This guide isn't about being a perfect mom." It has to do with being a good mother. To be the best for him, you must figure out what works for you.

Emma saw that she didn't have to go alone on this adventure as she held her infant near. Others who have been in her shoes knew that taking care of herself came before taking care of her child. She sensed that her doubts and anxieties were beginning to fade and were being replaced by a serene assurance that she would eventually find her way.

Emma read the notebook once more that night while her baby slept peacefully next to her. This time, instead of viewing it as a set of guidelines, she started to see it as an opportunity to establish her own pace and path. It served as a roadmap for a happier, healthier journey for both her and her unborn child. She was aware that her kid would develop with her as she gained courage, wisdom, and endurance; he would be fed by the affection, attention, and happiness they would experience together.

This was the beginning of Emma's motherhood tale, which was based on baby steps reinforced by straightforward but effective tactics and fortified by the knowledge she would eventually come to value and impart. As she and her child learned to get along, this was a journey that should be fully embraced day by day, rather than one that must be travelled flawlessly.

One of the most life-changing experiences is becoming a mother. A new chapter of excitement, expectation, and even anxiety begins the moment you find out you are expecting. The thought of having a life inside of you makes you want to do everything in your power to keep your kid and yourself healthy and happy. Setting the groundwork for a lifetime of well-being for both you and your kid is the goal of this journey, which goes beyond a nine-month schedule.

Welcome to *The Well Baby, Well Mom Guide*, a book created to guide you through one of the most life-changing experiences: becoming a mother. Since mother and child health are closely related, we hope that each chapter will help you build a foundation of well-being that supports you and your unborn child. There is nothing like this journey. It is full of happiness, learning, difficulties, and ongoing transformation. The journey of motherhood necessitates balance, flexibility, and, above all, self-compassion from the time you start making plans for a child until the time of delivery and beyond.

The fundamental tenet of this book is that mothers who put their health and well-being first create a foundation of strength and resilience that immediately helps their kids. Mothers require an equally supportive atmosphere that values their health, recognizes their emotional needs, and empowers them through every stage of their journey, just as newborns require love, care, and consistency to grow. These pages provide a thorough approach to wellness for both mother and child through insights, evidence-based recommendations, and useful resources.

To support this dual focus, *The Well Baby, Well Mom Guide* includes chapters on self-care, sleep, exercise, diet, and even marital support. It covers everything from physical health to emotional and mental wellness. Every section provides helpful guidance, knowledgeable analysis, and simple tactics that can be tailored to your particular way of living. The objective is to offer practical, powerful strategies that are easily modified to meet the constantly shifting needs of a new baby's life. In addition to these wellness techniques, you'll discover how to establish a supportive environment that upholds you both and provides stability and self-assurance even in the face of adversity.

Being a mother is more than a set of milestones or a never-ending to-do list. It's a period of significant personal development, exploration, and opportunity. How you approach every day, every choice you make, and every happy or challenging experience depends on your well-being. Research has indicated that the physical and mental well-being of a mother has a substantial impact on the development, resilience, and even emotional control of her child. In addition to taking care of yourself, you're also fostering the finest environment for your child's long-term well-being by embracing your wellness journey. Even if this path is frequently happy, it's equally critical to recognize the difficult times and allow oneself the freedom to ask for assistance, take breaks when necessary, and form support networks.

This book offers wellness advice as well as suggestions for bolstering your support systems. Creating a network of support, whether it be through friends, family, or a group of other mothers, can offer consolation, knowledge, and a feeling of oneness. Keep in mind that you are not supposed to handle everything by yourself. A healthy path for you and your child depends on accepting assistance, exchanging stories, and developing deep connections.

You'll find a combination of helpful resources and kind words of support in *The Well Baby, Well Mom Guide*, which will help you feel strong, competent, and taken care of. This book is intended to be a resource you can use when you require guidance, comfort, or simply some alone time. Consider it a toolkit that emphasizes sustainability, adaptability, and balance for both the expected and the unknown. Being healthy is about making decisions that will benefit you and your family in the long run, not about doing everything flawlessly.

As you prepare for this trip, remember that every action you take to improve your health is a gift to your future self, your child, your family, and yourself. Prioritizing well-being will provide a solid foundation that develops with you both through all of the ups and downs, achievements, and losses. We hope that this book will encourage you to embrace the fullness of motherhood, with all its joys and challenges, while fostering a healthy, meaningful life for both you and your child.

Together, let's set out on this road with compassion, purpose, and the understanding that by looking after yourself, you're also laying the finest possible foundation for your child's future.

# CHAPTER 1: A JOURNEY TO WELLNESS

Wellness is not merely the absence of illness; it's an active pursuit of physical, mental, and emotional health. Each person's journey to wellness is unique and involves identifying what truly nurtures our well-being. It asks us to cultivate habits that align with our needs. This process is ongoing, often nonlinear, requiring us to reevaluate our relationship with ourselves, our environment, and the practices that sustain our health.

Wellness is not just the absence of illness; it's an active pursuit of physical, mental, and emotional health that nurtures all aspects of our lives. The journey to wellness is highly personal and unique for each individual, as it requires us to identify what truly nourishes our well-being and to cultivate habits that align with these needs. This process is ongoing, often nonlinear, and asks us to examine and refine our relationship with ourselves, our environment, and the practices that support our best health.

The journey to wellness often begins with a commitment to self-awareness. Knowing where we stand—our strengths, limitations, and the sources of our physical or emotional discomfort—is essential for identifying what we need to feel balanced and fulfilled. Wellness also calls us to assess the factors that hinder or support our goals, from dietary habits to the quality of our relationships and even the impact of daily stressors. Building this awareness can mean looking at how we spend our time, the foods we consume, or the beliefs we hold about ourselves and our capabilities.

Achieving wellness often includes adopting physical practices, as bodily health is a key component. Whether it is exercise, a balanced diet, or adequate rest, physical health lays the foundation for energy, resilience, and mental clarity. Each of us has a unique physical makeup, so finding the right forms of movement and nutrition can require exploration and patience. For some, intense workouts provide stress relief, while others may benefit from more gentle activities like yoga or walking in nature. The goal is not perfection but rather developing sustainable habits that respect and nurture the body.

Emotional and mental wellness are equally crucial parts of the journey. These may involve mindfulness practices, therapy, or simply spending time with loved ones. Understanding and managing our thoughts and emotions enhances resilience, fosters positivity, and enables us to handle challenges gracefully. Wellness here means recognizing the importance of mental health and being proactive in addressing stress and negative patterns.

Cultivating a supportive social network also plays a significant role in well-being. Positive relationships provide a sense of belonging, reduce feelings of isolation, and enhance our emotional resilience. Taking time to nurture meaningful connections and setting healthy boundaries can transform how we experience daily interactions, adding joy, security, and empathy to our lives.

Finally, the journey to wellness involves flexibility and self-compassion. Life's demands shift and our understanding of wellness must adapt accordingly. Self-compassion allows us to navigate setbacks without harsh self-judgment, appreciating each small success as part of the greater journey. Wellness is a lifelong process, one in which progress may sometimes be slow but always enriching.

Wellness is about balance-finding harmony between our needs, goals, and the actions we take to support them. It is a journey of self-discovery and self-care, where every choice we make brings us closer to a life that is not just about surviving, but truly thriving.

## Understanding Maternal Health

Maternal health refers to women's health during pregnancy, childbirth, and the postpartum period. It encompasses the physical, mental, and social well-being of the mother, ensuring that she remains healthy throughout pregnancy, delivers safely, and recovers well afterwards. Maternal health is an essential public health concern, as it not only affects the mother but also has profound implications for the baby's health and development.

Maternal health encompasses the physical, mental, and emotional well-being of women during pregnancy, childbirth, and the postpartum period. This comprehensive field focuses on a mother's health before conception, throughout pregnancy, during labour and delivery, and after the birth of the child. Good maternal health is crucial not only for the well-being of mothers but also for the health and development of their infants. It is a critical public health issue, affecting families and communities on a wide scale, and demands attention to various aspects of healthcare, education, and policy.

Maternal health begins with prenatal care, which includes early and regular check-ups that allow healthcare providers to monitor both the mother's and the baby's health, address any issues as they arise, and provide essential health information. Early prenatal care can help detect and manage conditions such as gestational diabetes, preeclampsia, and infections that may pose risks to both mother and baby. Nutrition is a key focus during this period, as adequate intake of certain vitamins and minerals, including folic acid, iron, and calcium, is essential to reduce the risk of birth defects and other complications. Nutritional guidance during prenatal care also supports the mother's health, helping to prevent anaemia and maintain sufficient energy levels.

Childbirth and delivery are central events in the maternal health journey and require skilled care and monitoring to ensure the safety of both mother and baby. There are multiple options for childbirth, including vaginal delivery, cesarean section, and assisted delivery methods such as vacuum extraction or the use of forceps, and each has implications for maternal and infant health. The choice of delivery method is influenced by factors such as the health of the mother, the baby's position, and the presence of any complications. For example, a cesarean section may be necessary if there are risks that could make vaginal delivery unsafe. During labour and delivery, continuous monitoring helps healthcare providers quickly identify and respond to emergencies, such as fetal distress or maternal haemorrhage, reducing the risks of morbidity and mortality.

After childbirth, the postpartum period focuses on the mother's recovery and adjustment to new physical, mental, and emotional demands. Physically, this period involves recovery from the process of labour and, in cases of cesarean section, surgical healing. Postpartum care includes managing pain, monitoring for infection, and supporting the mother's general physical recovery. Mental health is a crucial component of postpartum care as well, given the prevalence of postpartum depression and anxiety, which can affect many mothers and impact their ability to care for their infants. Early identification and support for postpartum mental health are essential to ensure the well-being of both mother and child. Moreover, lactation support and guidance on infant care are provided to mothers during this time to help establish breastfeeding, which benefits both mother and child nutritionally and immunologically, and to promote secure infant care practices.

Maternal health, however, is often challenged by limited access to healthcare, particularly in low-resource settings where maternal mortality rates are highest. While advanced healthcare systems offer extensive maternal care, many regions globally lack the infrastructure, resources, and skilled personnel needed to support safe pregnancies and deliveries. Socioeconomic and cultural barriers also pose challenges, as poverty and a lack of education or healthcare literacy can prevent women from seeking or receiving timely care. In some regions, traditional practices or societal norms may limit women's access to healthcare, exacerbating the risks of complications and reducing maternal health outcomes.

Maternal mortality remains a global concern, with leading causes including haemorrhage, infections, high blood pressure disorders, and complications from unsafe abortions. These issues highlight the urgent need for improvements in maternal healthcare, especially in vulnerable populations. Globally, various initiatives aim to reduce maternal mortality and improve maternal health outcomes, including the United Nations' Sustainable Development Goals (SDGs), which call for significant reductions in maternal mortality rates by improving healthcare access and quality, addressing inequality, and enhancing healthcare infrastructure.

Preventive measures in maternal health include immunization, health education, and health policies that ensure access to quality maternal healthcare services. Vaccines, such as those for rubella and tetanus, are crucial in protecting both mothers and babies from preventable diseases that could otherwise have severe or fatal outcomes. Additionally, health education in communities encourages pregnant women to seek early and continuous prenatal care, teaches signs of potential complications, and promotes better nutritional and lifestyle choices. Policies focused on maternal health provide the necessary support for healthcare infrastructure, funding, and training for healthcare providers, which together work to reduce risks and promote better maternal and infant health outcomes.

Improving maternal health is not only a matter of individual well-being but also a broader social issue. A mother's health profoundly affects her family and community; when maternal health is compromised, the impact often extends to the health, education, and economic well-being of her children and family. As such, investments in maternal health yield broad, intergenerational benefits, creating healthier communities and reducing healthcare costs. Ensuring maternal health through adequate care, skilled support, and robust public health policies is foundational to a healthier, more sustainable society.

Maternal health is a complex and multifaceted issue that requires a holistic approach encompassing physical, mental, and social well-being. Ensuring that women receive the care, support, and resources they need before, during, and after pregnancy is crucial not only for the health of the mother but also for the well-being of her child and the future of society. By focusing on improving healthcare access, addressing social determinants, and educating women about maternal health, we can build healthier, stronger communities where mothers and babies thrive.

## The Importance of Prenatal Care

Parental care refers to any behaviour pattern in which a parent invests time or energy in feeding and protecting its offspring, it includes the provision of basic needs, showing affection and love, and any other behaviour that indicates concern for the child's welfare. Parental care could also be considered as any activity by a parent that contributes to increasing the fitness of its offspring. It can begin before birth with the building of a nest or den for the eggs or offspring. During reproduction, mothers can positively influence their developmental and survival chances by producing eggs that are as large and nutritious as possible or large live-born young. This aspect of brood care is the only one that is independent of behaviour; rather, it is a fundamental life history decision concerning the number and size of offspring. Nutrient supply to the eggs or developing juveniles is another aspect of parental care. After all, some offspring are so helpless after hatching or birth that their survival depends crucially on parental care. Whether and which form of parental care takes place depends on the ratio of the related benefits and costs. The benefits of care include positive effects on the survival, growth and reproductive success of the offspring. The somatic and environmental costs of parental care may be reflected in reduced survival, reduced fecundity in the next reproductive cycle and reduced fitness of the next set of offspring. The level of these costs depends strongly on current environmental conditions, but also parental conditions.

Parental care is essential for the physical, emotional, and social development of a child. It serves as the foundation for nurturing, protection, and support, playing a critical role in shaping a child's overall well-being and future success. Through parental care, children acquire the skills, values, and resilience needed to navigate life's challenges and build healthy relationships. The influence of parental care begins before birth and extends through adolescence, profoundly impacting a child's health, personality, and academic and social outcomes.

One of the primary roles of parental care is to ensure the child's physical health and safety. This care begins in pregnancy, with a mother's nutrition, health habits, and prenatal care directly impacting the developing fetus. A healthy prenatal environment contributes to normal fetal development, reducing risks of complications and ensuring that the child is born healthy. After birth, parental care includes providing adequate nutrition, shelter, healthcare, and physical protection. These necessities are essential for survival and healthy growth, enabling children to reach important developmental milestones. When parents are attentive to a child's health needs, the child is more likely to experience fewer illnesses, benefit from better cognitive development, and be equipped to excel in other areas of life.

Beyond physical health, parental care is crucial for emotional and psychological development. Children need consistent love, affection, and emotional support to develop a secure attachment and a strong sense of self. The emotional bond between parents and children provides a safe environment in which children can explore their surroundings, learn about themselves, and feel valued. A child who feels loved and secure is more likely to develop confidence, self-esteem, and resilience, all of which are key for positive mental health. Studies have shown that children who receive stable and nurturing care tend to experience fewer behavioural and emotional issues, show higher levels of social competence, and have healthier relationships. This secure attachment fosters empathy, cooperation, and the ability to manage emotions, which are fundamental traits for successful interactions in society.

Parental care also plays a pivotal role in cognitive and educational development. Parents introduce children to learning experiences, model language, and problem-solving behaviors, and provide the stimulation necessary for intellectual growth. From early infancy, parents who read to their children, engage in conversations, and introduce age-appropriate games and activities are helping develop their children's language skills, critical thinking, and creativity. These early interactions build a strong foundation for academic success, as children exposed to rich verbal interactions and varied learning experiences tend to develop better language, literacy, and mathematical skills. Active parental involvement in schooling, such as helping with homework and attending school events, reinforces the value of education and improves academic outcomes.

Social development is another area where parental care has a substantial impact. Children learn social skills primarily through observing and interacting with their parents. By modelling empathy, respect, and cooperation, parents help children learn how to form and maintain healthy relationships with others. Parental guidance in managing conflicts, making friends, and understanding social norms equips children with the tools they need to navigate social environments successfully. Positive parental role modelling helps children develop qualities like respect for others, patience, and honesty, which contribute to building meaningful connections throughout life.

Moreover, parental care contributes to a child's moral and ethical development. Parents are a child's first teachers, imparting values and helping children distinguish right from wrong. Through their actions and expectations, parents set boundaries that help children understand the importance of rules and respect for others. Children who receive guidance and support in developing a moral compass are more likely to grow up with a sense of accountability and an understanding of their role within their community. These values form the basis of responsible, ethical behaviour in adulthood, making children more likely to contribute positively to society.

In addition, parental care provides the foundation for resilience, teaching children how to cope with stress and adversity. Parents who provide a safe, stable, and supportive environment help their children build confidence in their ability to face challenges. When parents encourage problem-solving, show support during difficult times, and teach stress-management techniques, children develop a stronger sense of resilience and are better prepared to handle life's setbacks. Resilient children tend to experience better mental health and adapt more easily to changes and challenges, which are essential skills in an unpredictable world.

Parental care is essential to a child's holistic development. From physical health to emotional security, cognitive growth to social skills, the influence of caring, engaged parents is profound and far-reaching. Parents are not only the protectors and providers of their children but also their primary educators, role models, and sources of emotional support. By meeting these needs, parents lay the groundwork for their children to grow into well-rounded, healthy, and capable individuals. Parental care shapes children into compassionate, responsible adults, empowering them to contribute meaningfully to their communities and society at large.

## Nutrition Essentials for Expecting Moms

Nutrition during pregnancy is crucial for the health of both the mother and the developing baby, as it directly influences fetal growth, development, and the overall pregnancy experience. An expecting mother's diet must provide the necessary nutrients, vitamins, and minerals to support the increased demands on her body, as well as to contribute to a healthy pregnancy outcome. Among the essential nutrients are protein, iron, calcium, folic acid, and omega-3 fatty acids, each playing a specific role in maternal and fetal health.

Protein is fundamental during pregnancy as it supports fetal tissue growth, including the brain, and helps develop the mother's breast and uterine tissues. Pregnant women require increased protein intake, as it aids in the production of enzymes and hormones essential for fetal development. High-protein foods such as lean meats, poultry, fish, eggs, dairy products, and legumes are excellent sources. Protein also helps in maintaining blood sugar levels, which can reduce the risk of gestational diabetes.

Folic acid, a B vitamin, is essential from the very beginning of pregnancy, even before conception, as it plays a key role in preventing neural tube defects such as spina bifida. These birth defects occur early in pregnancy, often before a woman knows she is pregnant, making early folic acid intake crucial. Folic acid aids in the formation of the neural tube, which later develops into the baby's brain and spinal cord. It is recommended that women consume folic acid supplements or foods rich in folate, like dark leafy greens, legumes, citrus fruits, and fortified grains.

Iron is another critical nutrient because it supports the increased blood volume that occurs during pregnancy, which is necessary to supply oxygen to both the mother and baby. Iron deficiency anaemia is common during pregnancy and can lead to fatigue, weakened immunity, and, in severe cases, complications such as preterm delivery or low birth weight. To enhance iron absorption, iron-rich foods like lean meats, poultry, fish, and beans should be paired with foods high in vitamin C, such as oranges, strawberries, or bell peppers, which improve iron uptake. Expecting mothers may also benefit from iron supplements, though these should only be taken under medical supervision to avoid excess iron intake.

Calcium supports the development of the baby's bones, teeth, heart, muscles, and nervous system. Since fetal development places high demands on the mother's calcium stores, an insufficient calcium intake can lead to the depletion of the mother's bone density, as calcium is redirected from her bones to support the fetus. Dairy products are an excellent source of calcium, as are leafy green vegetables, almonds, and fortified plant milk. Pregnant women should aim for adequate calcium intake throughout pregnancy to protect both their bone health and that of their growing baby.

Omega-3 fatty acids, particularly DHA (docosahexaenoic acid), are essential for fetal brain and eye development. These fatty acids support the growth of brain cells and the formation of the retina, enhancing cognitive and visual function in the baby. Omega-3s can be found in fatty fish such as salmon, sardines, and trout, and in smaller amounts in plant-based sources like flaxseeds, chia seeds, and walnuts. DHA supplements derived from fish oil or algae are also available, but they should be taken with caution to avoid high levels of mercury and should be discussed with a healthcare provider.

Vitamin D is equally important as it works in tandem with calcium to support bone health and immune function. During pregnancy, vitamin D aids in the absorption of calcium, ensuring that both the mother and baby benefit from adequate levels. Sunlight exposure can help the body synthesize vitamin D, but it is also available in fortified dairy products, egg yolks, and fatty fish. In cases where vitamin D intake is insufficient, a healthcare provider may recommend a supplement.

Fibre is another important element of a pregnancy diet, as it helps manage digestion and reduces the likelihood of constipation, which is common during pregnancy. High-fiber foods include whole grains, fruits, vegetables, and legumes. Fibre also helps in maintaining stable blood sugar levels, which can prevent gestational diabetes. Staying hydrated is equally vital to support fibre intake, as well as for managing fluid retention and preventing urinary tract infections, which are more common during pregnancy.

Pregnant women should also be mindful of certain foods and beverages that may pose risks to maternal or fetal health. For instance, alcohol is strictly discouraged due to its potential to cause fetal alcohol syndrome, which can lead to physical, behavioural, and cognitive disabilities. Caffeine intake should be limited, as excessive caffeine has been associated with an increased risk of miscarriage and low birth weight; moderate amounts, generally under 200 mg per day (about one 12-ounce cup of coffee), are considered safe for most pregnant women. Foods high in mercury, such as shark, swordfish, and king mackerel, should be avoided as mercury exposure can affect fetal brain development. Pregnant women should also avoid undercooked or raw meats, eggs, and fish, as well as unpasteurized dairy products, as these can carry harmful bacteria like listeria and salmonella, which pose risks to both mother and baby.

In addition to individual nutrients, a balanced, varied diet is crucial to provide all the vitamins and minerals required during pregnancy. Whole grains, fruits, vegetables, lean proteins, and healthy fats should be included in daily meals to ensure comprehensive nutrition. Frequent, smaller meals throughout the day can help manage nausea, a common pregnancy symptom, and ensure steady energy levels. Ideally, expectant mothers should consult with a healthcare provider or nutritionist to create a personalized dietary plan that meets their specific needs and accounts for any pre-existing health conditions.

In summary, proper nutrition during pregnancy provides the essential building blocks for fetal growth and supports the health of the mother. With increased nutrient requirements, an expecting mother's diet should focus on protein, folic acid, iron, calcium, omega-3 fatty acids, vitamin D, and fibre while avoiding potentially harmful substances. A well-balanced diet and appropriate supplementation as recommended by healthcare professionals can significantly improve pregnancy outcomes and foster a healthy start for the newborn.

# CHAPTER 2: NURTURING MIND AND BODY

Nurturing the mind and body is a holistic approach to well-being that emphasizes the interconnection between mental and physical health. This integrated approach recognizes that caring for one's mental state has a profound impact on physical health, and vice versa. When one aspect of our well-being is neglected, it often affects the other. Nurturing both mind and body is essential for achieving optimal health, resilience, and fulfilment, and it involves developing habits and routines that address emotional, mental, and physical needs.

Mental nurturing begins with practices that promote emotional stability and cognitive clarity. This includes engaging in self-reflection, which allows individuals to understand their emotional patterns and triggers. By regularly taking time to reflect, whether through journaling, meditation, or quiet contemplation, one gains insight into areas of stress and happiness, leading to more intentional responses to daily challenges.

Meditation, in particular, is a widely practised technique that encourages mindfulness—a state of being fully present in the moment. This practice has been shown to reduce stress, enhance focus, and promote a greater sense of peace. Meditation helps calm the mind by slowing down the stream of thoughts, enabling individuals to experience a deeper sense of awareness and control over their emotions. Regular mindfulness practices not only foster mental clarity but also improve physical health by reducing stress hormones that contribute to conditions like high blood pressure, anxiety, and immune system deficiencies.

Emotional nurturing is another vital aspect of mental care. Emotions play a central role in how we perceive and respond to the world, and addressing them proactively can prevent mental exhaustion and burnout. Emotional intelligence, or the ability to recognize, understand, and manage emotions, is a valuable skill that enables people to navigate personal and social challenges more effectively. Nurturing emotional health requires engaging in activities that foster positive emotions, like connecting with loved ones, pursuing hobbies, and participating in creative or recreational outlets. Establishing a support network of friends, family, or support groups can provide valuable emotional resources, helping individuals feel understood and valued. When people have reliable support networks, they are more likely to manage stress effectively, experience higher life satisfaction, and maintain a positive outlook, all of which are fundamental to mental health.

Physical nurturing complements mental and emotional health by providing the body with the care and energy it needs to function optimally. Physical exercise is one of the most effective ways to nurture the body, as it strengthens muscles, improves cardiovascular health, and boosts mood by releasing endorphins—natural mood elevators. Regular exercise has been linked to a lower risk of chronic illnesses such as heart disease, diabetes, and obesity. Additionally, exercise plays a critical role in mental health by reducing symptoms of depression and anxiety, improving sleep quality, and increasing self-esteem. Physical nurturing also includes proper nutrition, which is foundational to sustaining energy levels, supporting cognitive function, and promoting immune health. A balanced diet rich in whole grains, fruits, vegetables, lean proteins, and healthy fats provides the essential nutrients the body needs for repair and maintenance. Certain foods, such as those rich in omega-3 fatty acids, antioxidants, and vitamins B and D, have been shown to support brain health and reduce inflammation, linking diet directly to cognitive and emotional well-being.

Rest and sleep are equally essential to nurturing both mind and body. Quality sleep allows the brain to consolidate memories, process emotions, and remove toxins, while also enabling the body to repair tissues, regulate hormones, and strengthen immunity. Lack of sleep can impair cognitive function, increase irritability, and raise stress levels, negatively impacting mental health. To ensure restorative sleep, establishing a consistent sleep routine, minimizing screen time before bed, and creating a comfortable sleep environment are crucial. Adequate sleep supports physical performance, enhances emotional resilience, and promotes sharper cognitive abilities, creating a stable foundation for overall wellness.

Nurturing the mind and body also includes managing stress effectively. Chronic stress, if unchecked, can lead to mental health issues like anxiety and depression, and it also has numerous negative effects on physical health, including increased inflammation, weakened immunity, and a higher risk of heart disease. Effective stress management techniques include practising deep breathing exercises, progressive muscle relaxation, and engaging in creative outlets such as art, music, or writing. These activities serve as both mental and physical outlets, reducing stress by promoting relaxation and allowing individuals to process emotions constructively. Regular breaks from work, spending time in nature, and participating in social activities also provide mental rest and improve mood. In recent years, "forest bathing," or spending time immersed in nature, has gained popularity for its stress-reducing benefits, as it encourages mindfulness and a sense of calm by connecting individuals to the natural environment. These strategies create a balanced approach to stress, preventing it from accumulating and leading to burnout.

Engaging the mind in stimulating activities is another important component of nurturing mental health. Activities like reading, puzzles, learning a new skill, or engaging in intellectually challenging conversations help keep the mind sharp, improve memory, and delay cognitive decline. Mental exercises stimulate neuroplasticity, the brain's ability to form new connections and pathways, which is vital for lifelong learning and adaptation. Intellectual engagement not only keeps the brain active but also promotes a sense of purpose and accomplishment, enhancing self-worth and motivation. This intellectual nurturing is particularly beneficial as it complements physical health practices, creating a well-rounded approach to wellness that involves lifelong learning and personal growth.

Self-care is a broader aspect of nurturing the mind and body that encompasses taking intentional time to recharge and engage in activities that bring joy and relaxation. Self-care routines vary from person to person and can include physical activities like yoga, pampering rituals like baths, or relaxation methods like reading or listening to music. The purpose of self-care is to give oneself permission to pause, which is particularly important in today's fast-paced society where burnout is common. Engaging in regular self-care activities reinforces self-compassion and respect for one's needs, contributing to a healthier mental state and a more resilient body.

Setting goals and fostering a sense of purpose is equally essential in nurturing the mind and body. Having clear, achievable goals gives individuals direction and motivation, which supports mental well-being by creating a sense of accomplishment and satisfaction. These goals do not need to be grand; they can be simple, like establishing a new hobby or improving physical fitness. The pursuit of goals fosters resilience, encouraging people to persevere through challenges and continue growing. By aligning daily actions with long-term aspirations, individuals experience greater fulfilment, which reinforces both mental and physical well-being.

Nurturing the mind and body is a comprehensive approach that requires attention to mental, emotional, and physical needs. Practices like mindfulness, emotional intelligence, regular exercise, balanced nutrition, quality sleep, and intellectual stimulation all contribute to holistic wellness. This approach to self-care creates a foundation for long-term health, resilience, and personal growth. By nurturing both the mind and body, individuals enhance their capacity to face life's challenges, leading to a more balanced, purposeful, and satisfying life. This balanced approach ultimately cultivates a state of harmony, where mental clarity and physical vitality support one another, resulting in optimal health and a heightened sense of well-being.

Mental wellness during pregnancy is essential for both the mother's well-being and the healthy development of the fetus. Pregnancy often brings a mix of emotions, hormonal shifts, and lifestyle changes, all of which can impact mental wellness. Maintaining emotional balance, managing stress, and cultivating resilience are key strategies for a positive pregnancy experience. A mentally well mother is better equipped to handle the physical demands of pregnancy and adapt to the transition into parenthood.

## Mental Wellness during Pregnancy

One of the key aspects of mental wellness during pregnancy is emotional regulation. The hormonal changes that occur can make a woman more susceptible to mood swings, irritability, and heightened sensitivity. Hormones such as estrogen and progesterone fluctuate considerably, affecting neurotransmitter levels and altering mood regulation. This is often exacerbated by the physical discomforts of pregnancy, such as nausea, fatigue, and body aches, which can lead to frustration and a sense of being overwhelmed. To manage these emotional shifts, it is helpful for expectant mothers to develop coping strategies, such as mindfulness meditation, journaling, and other forms of self-reflection. Mindfulness meditation helps increase awareness of one's emotions and reduces stress by promoting a sense of calm and presence. Journaling allows mothers to process and express their emotions privately, making it easier to understand and accept their feelings rather than suppressing or avoiding them.

Social support is another essential element of mental wellness during pregnancy. Having a reliable network of friends, family, or even support groups can provide comfort, reduce feelings of isolation, and help alleviate fears and concerns related to pregnancy and childbirth. Conversations with others who have experienced pregnancy can offer validation and practical advice, giving the mother a sense of reassurance. Social interactions stimulate the release of oxytocin, often called the "bonding hormone," which has natural stress-reducing properties. These interactions can make expectant mothers feel more connected and secure, allowing them to better manage the emotional demands of pregnancy. Additionally, professional support from a counsellor or therapist who specializes in prenatal care can provide essential guidance, helping mothers-to-be cope with any stress or anxieties that may arise. A therapist can also teach techniques like cognitive-behavioural strategies that empower women to reframe negative thoughts and respond more constructively to challenges.

Anxiety and worry are common experiences for many pregnant women and addressing these feelings is crucial for maintaining mental wellness. Pregnancy often brings a mix of excitement and concern, with worries about the baby's health, the mother's ability to handle childbirth, and fears about parenting. These concerns, while natural, can escalate into more significant anxieties if not managed well. To cope with anxiety, it can be helpful for expectant mothers to focus on evidence-based information and take control of the things within their power, such as attending regular prenatal appointments, learning about childbirth options, and preparing a support plan for after delivery. Mindfulness practices like deep breathing exercises and visualization can also help reduce anxiety by calming the nervous system and diverting focus from intrusive thoughts. Having a routine that incorporates relaxation techniques helps mitigate worry, making it easier to focus on the positive aspects of pregnancy rather than potential risks.

Physical wellness is deeply connected to mental wellness during pregnancy, as a healthy body fosters a healthy mind. Regular physical activity, approved by a healthcare provider, can significantly improve mood, reduce stress, and increase energy levels. Exercise stimulates the release of endorphins, hormones that create feelings of happiness and relaxation. Activities like walking, swimming, and prenatal yoga are gentle yet effective ways to stay active while minimizing physical strain. Prenatal yoga, in particular, combines physical movement with breath control and meditation, promoting both physical flexibility and mental clarity. Engaging in regular exercise also improves sleep, which is essential for mental well-being, as sleep disruptions during pregnancy can lead to increased irritability, anxiety, and mental fatigue.

Maintaining mental wellness during pregnancy also involves a strong emphasis on self-care. Pregnancy often requires adjustments in daily routines, and setting aside time for self-care can help create balance and reduce stress. This may include restful activities such as reading, listening to music, or taking warm baths, as well as creative outlets like painting or crafting. Self-care is about honouring one's needs and acknowledging the physical and emotional effort involved in pregnancy. By prioritizing relaxation and moments of enjoyment, expectant mothers give themselves permission to pause and recharge, which reinforces emotional resilience. Self-compassion, an integral part of self-care, encourages mothers to be kind to themselves, reducing the tendency to feel guilty or anxious over perceived shortcomings. This nurturing approach fosters a positive mental state and allows mothers to focus on the present moment, rather than worrying about unknowns.

Sleep is an essential factor for mental wellness during pregnancy, as it enables cognitive function, mood regulation, and physical recovery. Hormonal changes, physical discomfort, and anxiety can disrupt sleep, leading to exhaustion and irritability. Poor sleep can exacerbate stress and increase the risk of mental health issues like anxiety and depression. Developing a consistent sleep routine, such as establishing a regular bedtime, avoiding caffeine late in the day, and creating a relaxing pre-sleep ritual, can improve sleep quality. Additionally, practising relaxation techniques before bed, such as deep breathing, stretching, or guided visualization, can help calm the mind and prepare the body for rest. Good sleep hygiene is essential for cognitive clarity and emotional stability, creating a foundation for mental wellness throughout pregnancy.

Nutrition is another foundational aspect of mental wellness during pregnancy. A balanced diet not only supports fetal development but also stabilizes mood and energy levels, reducing irritability and fatigue. Nutrient-dense foods rich in omega-3 fatty acids, B vitamins, and antioxidants promote brain health, while complex carbohydrates and proteins help regulate blood sugar, preventing mood swings associated with energy dips. Consuming regular, balanced meals and staying hydrated are simple yet effective ways to maintain both physical and mental health during pregnancy. Nutritional habits have a direct impact on brain function and emotional well-being, reinforcing the mind-body connection that is so vital during this time.

An expectant mother's self-identity and sense of purpose can shift dramatically during pregnancy, sometimes leading to identity-related stress or uncertainty. Many women experience concerns about balancing their new role as mothers with other aspects of their identity, such as careers, hobbies, or social relationships. Processing these changes openly can prevent feelings of loss or resentment and help foster a healthy sense of self. Journaling about aspirations and fears, engaging in open conversations with a partner or friend, and setting intentions for personal goals post-pregnancy can ease the emotional adjustment. Cultivating a positive sense of self and self-efficacy during pregnancy helps mothers-to-be feel empowered and confident in their journey, which strengthens both mental wellness and overall resilience.

Finally, preparing for postpartum mental wellness is an essential aspect of mental health during pregnancy. Pregnancy can provide a period of reflection and planning, allowing mothers to prepare emotionally for the demands of parenthood. Familiarizing oneself with the signs of postpartum depression and anxiety, as well as having a postpartum support plan, can make it easier to seek help if needed. Postpartum preparation may involve arranging support from family and friends, planning for time off work, or connecting with mental health resources. Understanding that the postpartum period can bring emotional challenges, including hormonal changes and sleep deprivation, enables mothers to approach the experience with realistic expectations and a support system in place.

In conclusion, mental wellness during pregnancy is a multifaceted process involving emotional regulation, social support, anxiety management, physical wellness, self-care, sleep, nutrition, and identity exploration. Each of these elements contributes to a holistic approach that prepares mothers-to-be for the physical and emotional demands of pregnancy and parenthood. By nurturing mental wellness, expectant mothers are better equipped to handle the changes and challenges that arise, benefiting not only their health but also that of their growing child. This balanced approach supports a positive pregnancy experience, enabling mothers to approach their journey with confidence, resilience, and inner peace.

## Stress Management Techniques

Managing stress during and after childbirth is essential to ensure the health and well-being of both the mother and the newborn. The period surrounding childbirth is often filled with intense emotions, physical exhaustion, and a variety of new responsibilities, making stress management particularly crucial. Effective stress management during this time helps mothers adapt to the physical demands of birth and postpartum recovery while adjusting emotionally to the role of parenthood. Mothers who incorporate stress-relief techniques can experience a more positive birth experience, enhanced emotional resilience, and improved long-term mental wellness.

One of the primary stress management techniques during childbirth is focused breathing.

Controlled breathing exercises provide an immediate sense of calm, helping to regulate the nervous system and alleviate tension in the body. During labour, deep and rhythmic breathing can be used to maintain focus and manage the pain associated with contractions. Techniques such as slow breathing, where one inhales deeply for a count of four, holds the breath for a few seconds and then exhales slowly, encourage relaxation and help mothers stay present. Practising these breathing exercises before labour begins allows them to become second nature, providing a steadying anchor when labour pains intensify. Additionally, certain methods like Lamaze breathing focus on providing a structured breathing pattern that allows mothers to work with their body's natural rhythms, further minimizing stress and pain.

Support from a partner, doula, or birth coach is also essential in managing stress during childbirth. Having someone nearby who can offer encouragement, reassurance, and practical support creates a sense of safety and reduces feelings of isolation during labour. A supportive birth team, including compassionate medical staff, can help ease any fears or anxieties a mother may have, ensuring she feels understood and cared for. Emotional support reduces stress hormones like cortisol, promoting a more positive and empowered birth experience. Doulas, specifically trained to support mothers during labour, use a variety of comfort measures, such as massage, guidance through breathing exercises, and affirmations, to help mothers stay calm and focused. Knowing that there is a trusted support system can greatly alleviate anticipatory stress and create a supportive environment that encourages relaxation.

Visualization is another technique mothers can use during labour to manage stress and maintain a positive focus. Visualization involves creating a mental image of a peaceful place, a cherished memory, or an encouraging outcome, which helps divert attention from discomfort and fear. By mentally immersing themselves in calming or empowering imagery, mothers can reduce their perception of pain and foster a positive mindset. Visualization can be paired with affirmations, such as mentally repeating empowering phrases like "I am strong" or "I can do this," which reinforces self-confidence and reduces stress. Visualization and affirmations not only provide a mental distraction from labour pains but also encourage an attitude of resilience and acceptance of the birthing process, making it easier to navigate the physical challenges of labour.

After childbirth, rest and recovery become central to stress management, as the physical strain of birth and the demands of caring for a newborn can quickly lead to exhaustion. Rest, however, is often disrupted by the needs of a newborn, which makes finding moments of relaxation all the more essential. New mothers benefit from taking short naps when the baby sleeps, using comfortable positions for breastfeeding, and creating a relaxing sleep environment whenever possible. Postpartum rest improves mood, reduces irritability, and promotes healing, making it easier to manage stress. When adequate sleep is challenging to achieve, other relaxation methods like gentle stretching, deep breathing exercises, or listening to calming music can offer moments of reprieve, even if only briefly. Allowing oneself to prioritize rest helps mothers maintain their energy levels, preventing burnout and supporting physical recovery.

Social support is crucial during the postpartum period, as the first weeks after birth are often filled with a range of emotions, from joy and excitement to doubt and fatigue. Talking with friends, family members, or fellow new parents offers a valuable opportunity to share experiences and seek advice, reducing the sense of isolation that can accompany the early days of parenthood. For many, connecting with a supportive group, whether in person or through online communities, provides a sense of solidarity and shared understanding. Postpartum support groups provide an environment where mothers can openly discuss their experiences, receive encouragement, and learn practical coping strategies. Knowing that others are navigating similar challenges often provides comfort and reassurance, reducing the burden of self-doubt and stress. Additionally, family members or friends can help with practical tasks, such as cooking or running errands, allowing new parents more time to rest and bond with their baby.

Time management skills are essential during the postpartum period to help new mothers balance their responsibilities and reduce feelings of overwhelm. The routine of caring for a newborn is unpredictable and demanding, often requiring frequent feedings, diaper changes, and soothing. By organizing daily tasks and setting realistic expectations, mothers can better manage their time and prevent stress from accumulating. Setting aside small blocks of time for self-care activities, such as a short walk or a moment to enjoy a meal, provides essential breaks from the continuous demands of parenthood. Creating a flexible schedule that prioritizes both the baby's needs and the mother's well-being encourages a balanced approach to postpartum life. If possible, delegating tasks or setting up a rotating schedule with a partner can provide some relief, ensuring that the mother has designated moments for rest and recovery.

Mindfulness practices are effective for stress relief and emotional regulation during the postpartum period. Practising mindfulness helps mothers cultivate awareness of the present moment, reducing the impact of anxious thoughts or worries about the future. When feelings of self-doubt or overwhelm arise, mindfulness encourages mothers to observe their thoughts without judgment, allowing them to process emotions calmly and constructively. Techniques such as mindful breathing or grounding exercises help stabilize the mind, creating a sense of calm that makes it easier to respond to stressful situations with patience and clarity. By incorporating mindfulness into their daily routine, new mothers can better manage the emotional ups and downs of early parenthood and maintain a healthy mental state.

Self-compassion is another important technique in managing postpartum stress. New mothers often face high expectations, both from themselves and society, regarding parenting, physical recovery, and managing household responsibilities. Practising self-compassion involves treating oneself with kindness and understanding, especially in moments of perceived inadequacy or struggle. By acknowledging that parenthood is a learning process and that it is okay to make mistakes, mothers can reduce self-imposed stress and guilt. Self-compassionate attitudes promote mental wellness, reducing anxiety and encouraging a balanced perspective on the challenges of parenthood. Allowing oneself the space to rest and seek help, when needed, is an integral part of self-compassion and ultimately benefits both the mother and her child by fostering a positive and supportive mindset.

Light exercise, as permitted by a healthcare provider, can be a valuable way to manage postpartum stress. Gentle forms of exercise, such as walking, postpartum yoga, or stretching, help reduce muscle tension, improve circulation, and release endorphins, which are natural mood enhancers. Exercise also provides mothers with a sense of accomplishment and routine, creating a structured activity that helps alleviate stress and promote physical recovery. Yoga, in particular, combines gentle movement with breath control and mindfulness, which improves both physical flexibility and mental clarity. By integrating light exercise into daily life, mothers can gradually restore their strength and energy levels, supporting both physical and emotional well-being.

Good nutrition is essential for managing stress and maintaining energy during the postpartum period. A balanced diet that includes protein, complex carbohydrates, healthy fats, and a variety of fruits and vegetables supports the body's recovery and provides sustained energy. Hydration is also key, especially for breastfeeding mothers, as dehydration can contribute to fatigue and mood swings. Nutrient-dense foods such as leafy greens, whole grains, lean proteins, and omega-3-rich foods provide essential vitamins and minerals that support mental wellness and energy levels. Proper nutrition reduces physical stress on the body and supports the immune system, enhancing resilience and promoting a more positive postpartum experience.

Postpartum mental health support is another critical component of stress management, as some women experience postpartum depression or anxiety following childbirth. Recognizing early signs of postpartum depression, such as persistent sadness, irritability, or overwhelming fatigue, is essential for seeking timely help. Therapy, counselling, or support groups offer valuable resources for mothers experiencing mental health challenges. Professional support provides a safe space to discuss emotions and receive guidance on coping strategies. Learning and implementing techniques such as cognitive-behavioural therapy (CBT) can help mothers reframe negative thoughts and build resilience, while therapy offers a platform for exploring complex emotions and navigating the transition to parenthood. Access to mental health resources empowers mothers to manage stress proactively and fosters long-term well-being.

Stress management during and after childbirth involves a range of techniques that address physical, emotional, and practical needs. From focused breathing and visualization during labour to self-care practices and social support in the postpartum period, these techniques help mothers navigate the physical and emotional demands of parenthood. Practising mindfulness, self-compassion, good nutrition, and light exercise also contribute to a balanced approach to stress management, enabling mothers to recover and adapt with resilience. By incorporating these techniques into their daily lives, new mothers can foster a positive, supported, and empowered experience during this transformative time.

## The Role of Exercise and Movement

Exercise and movement play a crucial role in supporting the health and well-being of expecting and postpartum mothers, contributing to both physical and mental wellness. Before birth, physical activity prepares the body for the demands of pregnancy, labour, and delivery, enhancing flexibility, strength, and stamina. After childbirth, exercise supports postpartum recovery, helps restore physical function, and aids in managing emotional well-being. Properly tailored exercise routines before and after birth contribute to maternal health in unique ways, with each stage requiring specific considerations.

During pregnancy, exercise is essential for maintaining cardiovascular fitness, which supports circulation and oxygen delivery to both the mother and the developing baby. Cardiovascular exercises such as walking, swimming, and low-impact aerobics help maintain endurance, strengthen the heart, and support overall energy levels. These activities are particularly beneficial as they increase lung capacity and help regulate blood pressure, which reduces the risk of pregnancy-related hypertension. Maintaining cardiovascular fitness can also mitigate common discomforts associated with pregnancy, such as fatigue, shortness of breath, and poor circulation. Expecting mothers often find that regular cardiovascular activity improves sleep quality, reduces stress, and enhances mood, contributing to a positive pregnancy experience.

Strength training is another vital aspect of exercise during pregnancy, providing the muscle tone and stability needed to support the added weight and changing body dynamics. As the baby grows, the mother's centre of gravity shifts, placing increased strain on the back, hips, and pelvis. Strengthening core muscles, including the back, abdominal, and pelvic muscles, helps to support these areas and reduces discomfort. Exercises such as squats, lunges, and modified planks target these muscle groups while enhancing stability and balance. Strong muscles are better equipped to support the additional weight of pregnancy, reducing strain on joints and lowering the risk of injuries like back pain or pelvic discomfort. Strength training during pregnancy also prepares the body for labour, as toned muscles can better support prolonged physical exertion and facilitate easier movement during childbirth.

Flexibility exercises, such as those practised in prenatal yoga or stretching routines, are beneficial for maintaining a full range of motion and relieving tension in muscles and joints. Pregnancy often creates tension in the hips, lower back, and shoulders due to postural changes and added weight. Gentle stretching helps relieve these discomforts, encouraging better posture and alignment as the body adapts to pregnancy. Yoga, in particular, incorporates both stretching and strength-building movements, making it ideal for expecting mothers. Prenatal yoga also teaches valuable breathing techniques that can be used during labour to manage pain and anxiety. By maintaining flexibility, expecting mothers improve circulation and reduce stiffness, allowing for a more comfortable pregnancy and better physical mobility.

The mental benefits of exercise during pregnancy are also significant, as physical activity promotes the release of endorphins, the body's natural mood enhancers. Pregnancy can be a time of heightened emotions, with hormonal changes contributing to mood swings, anxiety, and stress. Exercise provides a natural means of managing these emotional fluctuations, fostering feelings of happiness and calm. Activities that incorporate mindfulness, such as yoga and walking, further reduce stress by encouraging a focus on the present moment. Mental well-being during pregnancy is critical for both the mother and baby, as high-stress levels can impact fetal development. By incorporating exercise, mothers create a stable foundation for a healthy emotional state, which also promotes bonding with the baby.

After childbirth, exercise remains essential for supporting the mother's recovery, helping to restore strength and stamina, and managing physical and emotional changes associated with the postpartum period. The initial weeks after birth require a gentle approach to movement, as the body is healing from delivery. Walking is often recommended as the first form of postpartum exercise due to its low impact and accessibility. Walking allows new mothers to reintroduce movement gradually, promoting circulation and preventing blood clots without placing stress on healing muscles or joints. Regular short walks can alleviate stiffness and improve energy levels, supporting the body's transition from rest to light activity.

As the mother's body begins to heal, gentle core-strengthening exercises become important for rebuilding abdominal and pelvic muscles that may have weakened during pregnancy and delivery. Diastasis recti, a common condition in which the abdominal muscles separate during pregnancy, can benefit from targeted exercises that strengthen the core without exacerbating the separation. Movements such as pelvic tilts, bridge lifts, and modified crunches are typically safe and effective, helping to gradually close the gap in the abdominal wall. Rebuilding core strength supports posture, reduces lower back pain, and contributes to a stable foundation for more advanced movements. Strong pelvic muscles also aid in bladder control and reduce the risk of pelvic organ prolapse, which can be a concern after childbirth.

Strength training for the upper and lower body is also valuable during the postpartum period. New mothers often find themselves lifting and carrying their baby frequently, which can place additional stress on the arms, shoulders, and back. Strengthening exercises, such as gentle bicep curls, shoulder presses, and leg lifts, help mothers build endurance for these new physical demands. Postpartum exercise routines that focus on functional movements—such as squats and lunges—improve daily mobility and reduce fatigue associated with caring for an infant. These exercises are particularly helpful in preventing injuries related to repetitive motions and improper lifting techniques, allowing mothers to handle the physical demands of childcare more comfortably.

Flexibility and relaxation exercises continue to offer benefits in the postpartum period, helping mothers reduce muscle tension, improve posture, and relax. Stretching movements that focus on the back, shoulders, and legs can relieve tension accumulated from prolonged sitting or holding the baby. Postnatal yoga is an excellent choice for postpartum flexibility, as it includes gentle stretching, deep breathing, and relaxation techniques. Yoga also encourages mothers to connect with their bodies mindfully, helping them to regain confidence and foster self-compassion as they adjust to the changes brought about by childbirth. These exercises allow mothers to listen to their body's cues, honouring the healing process and rebuilding a positive self-image.

Mental well-being is another area where exercise plays a critical role in the postpartum period, as it helps manage stress, anxiety, and depression. Postpartum depression and anxiety are common, affecting up to one in seven women. Exercise has been shown to reduce symptoms of depression by releasing endorphins and improving mood. The sense of accomplishment that comes with regular physical activity fosters confidence, helping mothers feel more in control of their health and recovery. Activities like yoga, walking, and swimming are particularly effective in promoting relaxation and mental clarity, providing new mothers with a way to recharge emotionally. Social forms of exercise, such as joining a postpartum yoga class or walking group, allow mothers to connect with others in similar situations, reducing feelings of isolation and fostering a supportive community.

Another important aspect of postpartum exercise is its effect on energy levels and physical endurance, both of which are often challenged by the demands of caring for a newborn. Physical activity helps new mothers regulate their sleep patterns and boosts energy by increasing circulation and metabolism. Gentle exercise during the day contributes to more restful sleep, even if the duration of sleep is limited by the baby's needs. Improved energy levels enable mothers to manage the physical demands of early parenthood with greater ease, reducing the fatigue that can contribute to stress and irritability. As mothers regain strength and stamina, they are better equipped to handle the lifting, bending, and movement involved in caring for a baby.

For mothers who are breastfeeding, exercise offers additional benefits. Regular, moderate exercise has been shown to support lactation by improving blood flow and supporting hormonal balance, which is essential for milk production. Engaging in physical activity does not negatively impact the quantity or quality of breast milk, and it may even provide a stress-relieving outlet that enhances the mother's sense of well-being. However, hydration is particularly important for breastfeeding mothers who exercise, as both breastfeeding and physical activity require adequate fluid intake. Staying hydrated ensures that the body has the resources it needs to produce milk and maintain energy levels, making it an important consideration for active new mothers.

Exercise and movement foster maternal health before and after birth. During pregnancy, regular cardiovascular activity, strength training, and flexibility exercises prepare the body for labour, support mental well-being, and improve physical comfort. Postpartum exercise supports recovery by rebuilding strength and flexibility, enhancing energy levels, and reducing symptoms of postpartum depression and anxiety. By incorporating physical activity suited to each stage of the maternal journey, mothers can navigate pregnancy and postpartum recovery with greater resilience and confidence, ultimately enhancing their overall health and quality of life.

# CHAPTER 3: CREATING A HEALTHY ENVIRONMENT

Creating a healthy environment before and after birth is essential for the well-being of both the mother and baby, setting the foundation for a supportive and nurturing atmosphere. A healthy environment considers physical, emotional, and social factors, each of which plays a crucial role in promoting maternal and infant health. By proactively preparing the home and social environment, expecting and new parents can reduce stress, encourage bonding, and foster a sense of security and comfort.

Before birth, creating a healthy environment begins with preparing the home for the arrival of a newborn. This preparation includes ensuring cleanliness, organization, and safety in all areas of the home where the baby will spend time. One of the first steps is to designate a sleeping area that is quiet, well-ventilated, and comfortable for both mother and baby. Many parents choose to set up a crib or bassinet in the same room, which allows for easy nighttime feeding and monitoring. The baby's sleeping environment should be free of clutter, with a firm mattress and no loose bedding or soft toys, to reduce the risk of sudden infant death syndrome (SIDS). Keeping the temperature in the room between 68–72°F is generally recommended for newborns, as this range helps maintain a comfortable and safe sleeping temperature.

Cleanliness in the home environment is also important to minimize exposure to allergens and potential irritants, which can impact the health of both mother and child. Regular dusting, vacuuming, and cleaning surfaces with mild, non-toxic cleaners help reduce exposure to allergens and airborne particles that could affect respiratory health. The use of natural or eco-friendly cleaning products can be beneficial, as they tend to be free from harsh chemicals that may be unsafe for infants. Expecting mothers should avoid exposure to strong chemicals or fumes that could be harmful during pregnancy, opting instead for safer alternatives. Indoor plants are a good addition to the home, as they help purify the air by absorbing pollutants and increasing oxygen levels, making the space feel fresher and cleaner.

Nutrition is another critical aspect of creating a healthy prenatal environment. Stocking the kitchen with nutrient-dense foods, such as fruits, vegetables, whole grains, and lean proteins, ensures that both mother and baby receive essential vitamins and minerals. An emphasis on foods rich in folic acid, iron, calcium, and omega-3 fatty acids supports fetal development and maternal health. Drinking ample water and minimizing processed foods also contribute to an overall healthy dietary environment, which can positively affect mood and energy levels. Preparing meals or freezing healthy snacks in advance can help during the early postpartum period when energy is low, and time is limited. These prepared meals ensure that nutritious options are readily available, allowing new mothers to focus on recovery and bonding with the baby.

The emotional environment in the home is equally important and is shaped by the mental well-being of the expecting parents. Pregnancy and early parenthood are often accompanied by intense emotions, making it essential to cultivate a supportive and low-stress atmosphere. Practising open communication, addressing fears or anxieties, and seeking social or professional support when needed are all ways to reduce emotional tension and promote harmony within the household. Creating a calm and peaceful environment includes establishing a routine that incorporates self-care, relaxation, and mindful activities. Soft lighting, calming music, and designated quiet spaces can all contribute to a tranquil atmosphere, providing areas where the mother can rest, meditate, or practice breathing exercises that promote relaxation. By nurturing mental wellness, parents build a stable foundation for coping with the upcoming changes of parenthood.

After birth, maintaining a healthy physical environment becomes essential as the newborn adapts to life outside the womb. Keeping the home clean and well-organized continues to be important, as babies have developing immune systems and are more susceptible to infections. Daily tidying, washing the baby's clothes and bedding with mild, fragrance-free detergents, and ensuring that feeding, diapering, and bathing supplies are readily accessible all help to create a functional and hygienic environment. Limiting exposure to screens and loud noises also promotes a calm setting, allowing the baby to adjust to the outside world in a comforting and soothing atmosphere. Soft, warm lighting is preferable in the nursery or sleeping area, as it can be more calming for both mother and baby during nighttime feedings or diaper changes.

Nutrition and hydration remain central to the mother's recovery and breastfeeding (if she chooses to breastfeed), as these aspects directly impact her physical and mental well-being. Maintaining a balanced diet with adequate hydration supports the mother's energy levels and helps her body heal. For breastfeeding mothers, consuming foods that provide calcium, iron, and protein is essential, as these nutrients support milk production and overall health. Additionally, eating a variety of fresh, nutrient-dense foods improves the quality of breast milk, providing essential nutrients to the baby. The presence of nutritious snacks and meals within the home creates an environment that encourages healthy eating habits, supporting both mother and child in the postpartum phase.

The social environment is also crucial for new parents, as social support can significantly impact emotional health and stress levels. Friends, family members, and community groups can offer practical help, such as meal preparation, babysitting, or assisting with household chores, allowing new parents more time to bond with their baby. Emotional support from a partner, family, or friends provides new mothers with a sense of security and reassurance, helping them navigate the challenges of postpartum recovery and caregiving. When friends or family offer support, parents can take short breaks or rest, which is essential for managing the physical demands of caring for a newborn. Support groups for new mothers also create a space where shared experiences and advice can be exchanged, helping mothers feel less isolated and more understood.

Creating a nurturing space for bonding and development in the home environment fosters a strong connection between mother and child. Incorporating skin-to-skin contact, cuddling, and soft, reassuring voices into daily interactions encourages emotional bonding and stimulates the baby's senses. Designating a comfortable space for bonding activities, such as feeding or reading to the baby, allows parents to establish a routine that nurtures their connection. Gentle activities like baby massage or tummy time provide sensory stimulation that supports the baby's physical and cognitive development, creating a safe and engaging environment that promotes growth and exploration. Maintaining a calm and predictable atmosphere in the home helps babies feel secure, which contributes to healthy emotional development and a sense of trust between the baby and caregiver.

Physical exercise in the postpartum period, such as gentle stretching or walking, is another way to create a balanced environment that supports the mother's recovery. Engaging in light physical activity can be uplifting, relieve muscle tension, and help regulate mood by releasing endorphins. Postpartum exercise helps mothers gradually rebuild strength, maintain flexibility, and increase energy levels. A designated area in the home for postpartum exercises, such as yoga or Pilates, provides a dedicated space for self-care and encourages a balanced routine. By taking time to exercise, even if only for a few minutes each day, mothers create a positive and supportive environment for their own mental and physical health, which, in turn, benefits their interactions with the baby.

Safety remains a priority in the home environment after birth, as babies begin to explore and grow rapidly. Childproofing the home involves securing furniture, covering electrical outlets, and ensuring that small objects or potentially hazardous items are out of reach. Installing smoke and carbon monoxide detectors, maintaining safe water temperatures, and using safe sleep practices further contribute to a protective environment. As the baby grows, having a safe, clean, and hazard-free space for exploration and play becomes important for development. Creating a child-friendly space where the baby can explore, play, and learn supports physical and cognitive growth, laying the foundation for healthy habits and a safe environment.

Creating a sustainable environment within the home can also support a family's health before and after birth. Simple actions like reducing single-use plastics, choosing eco-friendly products, and minimizing exposure to chemicals promote a healthier space. Opting for non-toxic baby products, from toys to skincare, ensures that the baby is exposed to safer materials. Sustainable choices also benefit the household's overall well-being, reducing the presence of toxins that can impact air quality and health. Additionally, these practices often contribute to a cleaner, more organized living space, further fostering a healthy and welcoming environment.

The mental environment after birth is another key element in creating a positive home environment for both mother and child. New mothers may experience a range of emotions, from joy to anxiety, and some may face postpartum depression. Prioritizing mental health through self-compassion, mindfulness, and, if needed, seeking professional support helps mothers process these emotions constructively. Creating a mental environment that allows time for self-care, reflection, and relaxation supports emotional stability, which enhances the mother's ability to connect with and care for her baby. Mindfulness practices such as meditation or deep breathing exercises are valuable for centring oneself amidst the demands of new parenthood, creating a sense of peace and presence that extends to the family environment.

Creating a healthy environment before and after birth involves preparing a safe, clean, and supportive physical space; fostering an emotionally nurturing atmosphere; and prioritizing the mental well-being of both mother and baby. By addressing these components, parents can create a balanced, healthy, and enriching environment that promotes growth, connection, and a smooth transition into parenthood. Establishing these practices ensures that the home is a space where both the mother and baby can thrive, setting the foundation for lifelong well-being and a positive family experience.

## Safe and Healthy Home Practices

Safe and healthy home practices before and after birth play an essential role in creating a secure and nurturing environment for both the mother and the newborn. These practices include maintaining physical cleanliness, ensuring mental well-being, organizing the home, and childproofing spaces to meet the needs of a growing family. A safe home environment allows expecting parents to feel prepared and ensures that new mothers and their babies experience comfort, stability, and protection from potential hazards. Additionally, such an environment supports the health of both mother and child by minimizing exposure to allergens, pollutants, and safety risks.

Before birth, preparing the home begins with creating a clean and organized space. Regular cleaning helps to reduce allergens, dust, and mould that may affect respiratory health, particularly for a pregnant mother whose immune system is often more sensitive. Using mild, non-toxic cleaners is ideal, as strong chemicals can pose risks to both the mother and developing baby. Natural cleaning agents, such as vinegar, baking soda, and castile soap, offer safe and effective alternatives that avoid exposure to toxic chemicals. Special attention should be given to areas where the baby will spend most of their time, including the nursery, sleeping area, and any shared family spaces. Expecting parents might consider investing in a high-quality vacuum with a HEPA filter to capture fine particles, as well as regularly washing linens, curtains, and soft furnishings. Adequate ventilation is also essential; opening windows and using an air purifier can help improve indoor air quality by reducing the concentration of pollutants.

Organizing the home before birth can make a significant difference in reducing stress and preparing for the newborn's arrival. Setting up designated areas for baby essentials, such as diapers, clothes, and feeding supplies, ensures that needed items are always within reach. Organizing these items in clearly labelled containers or storage spaces helps create a sense of order and minimizes confusion during the early, often sleep-deprived days of parenting. Many parents find it helpful to create a diapering station with essentials in one convenient spot, ideally near the baby's sleeping area, to make nighttime changes as smooth as possible. Similarly, setting up a comfortable feeding area, with a supportive chair and necessary supplies like burp cloths and blankets, allows for a peaceful and enjoyable feeding experience. By organizing items in advance, parents create a functional and supportive environment that eases the transition into the postpartum period.

Maintaining a safe home environment also means considering aspects of mental and emotional well-being. Pregnancy and early parenthood are times of intense physical and emotional demands, and a supportive home atmosphere can be a valuable source of comfort and stability. Creating a calm and peaceful environment, free from excessive noise or stress, can help both parents and the baby feel more relaxed. Setting aside a quiet space for relaxation, meditation, or even just resting, encourages the expecting mother to take regular breaks and stay attuned to her emotional health. This area can include comfortable seating, soft lighting, and perhaps soothing music to promote relaxation. Taking time for self-care activities, even if only for a few minutes each day, can be beneficial in maintaining mental well-being and reducing stress levels. Many parents find that the addition of calming scents, such as lavender or chamomile, can help set a soothing tone in the home and encourage a peaceful state of mind.

As the pregnancy progresses, focusing on childproofing the home becomes important, especially as the baby grows and begins to explore their surroundings. Childproofing before the baby's arrival allows parents to gradually implement safety measures and ensure that all potential hazards are addressed. In the nursery or baby's sleep space, ensure that the crib or bassinet meets safety standards, with a firm mattress and no loose bedding or soft toys that could pose suffocation risks. Installing smoke detectors and carbon monoxide detectors in key areas of the home adds a layer of protection, as does keeping fire extinguishers in accessible locations, such as the kitchen. Electrical outlets should be covered, and cords should be safely out of reach to prevent accidents. As the baby becomes more mobile, further adjustments will be needed, including securing furniture, using cabinet locks, and ensuring that small items, which pose choking hazards, are stored out of reach.

After birth, maintaining a clean, organized, and secure home environment remains essential, with additional focus on hygiene and convenience. With the mother recovering and the baby adjusting to the world outside the womb, cleanliness takes on renewed importance. Regular hand-washing and sanitizing surfaces, especially in areas where the baby spends time, can help minimize the spread of germs. Cleaning feeding bottles, pacifiers, and any toys the baby might put in their mouth is also important, as infants have developing immune systems and are more vulnerable to infections. Using a designated cleaning area for baby items, separate from other household cleaning tasks, adds an extra layer of sanitation. Creating a routine for laundering the baby's clothing and bedding with gentle, fragrance-free detergents further supports a clean environment, reducing the risk of irritation or allergic reactions.

Safety considerations become even more focused in the early postpartum period, as new parents adjust to caring for their newborn's needs. A safe sleep environment is a priority, and parents should follow guidelines for safe infant sleep practices. The baby should sleep on their back on a firm surface, without soft bedding or pillows, to reduce the risk of sudden infant death syndrome (SIDS). It is also beneficial to keep the baby's sleep area in the same room as the parents during the first few months, which allows for easy monitoring and reduces the risk of accidental suffocation. Swaddling can provide comfort and security for the baby, but parents should be mindful to swaddle safely, allowing room for hip movement to prevent hip dysplasia and ensuring that the swaddle is not too tight around the chest.

Postpartum nutrition is another crucial aspect of maintaining a healthy home environment, supporting the mother's recovery and, if applicable, breastfeeding needs. Having nutritious meals and snacks prepared and available in the home ensures that the mother has access to essential nutrients, even when time and energy are limited. Foods rich in iron, protein, calcium, and vitamins are especially beneficial, aiding in the body's healing process and supporting milk production. Many families find it helpful to stock the kitchen with simple, easy-to-prepare foods that require minimal effort, as well as ample water to stay hydrated, especially during breastfeeding. Family members or friends may also assist by preparing meals or organizing meal deliveries, further supporting the mother's nutritional needs and reducing stress during this demanding period.

Mental well-being is a cornerstone of a healthy postpartum environment. Having a strong support network, open lines of communication, and access to emotional support can help mothers cope with the psychological demands of early parenthood. The postpartum period can bring about intense emotions, ranging from joy and bonding to anxiety, fatigue, and even depression. Creating an environment that allows space for these emotions to be acknowledged and processed is essential. Partners, friends, or family members can support this process by offering empathy, encouragement, and practical help. Joining support groups or connecting with other parents can also provide reassurance and a sense of community, helping new mothers feel understood and less isolated. For mothers experiencing symptoms of postpartum depression, seeking professional support from a counsellor or therapist can be a valuable resource, and having a safe, supportive home environment encourages reaching out for help when needed.

Exercise though approached gently, can also contribute to a healthy environment, helping mothers regain physical strength and mental clarity. Light postpartum exercises, such as walking or gentle stretching, promote circulation and relieve muscle tension. Creating a space for short exercise routines within the home, even if just a small area with a mat or comfortable flooring, allows the mother to incorporate movement into her day as she feels ready. Physical activity, combined with adequate rest and a balanced diet, contributes to a mother's overall sense of well-being and can improve her ability to manage the physical demands of caring for a newborn.

As the baby grows and becomes more curious about their surroundings, additional safety precautions are needed. Childproofing measures should evolve in response to the baby's increasing mobility and curiosity, ensuring that potentially dangerous items are out of reach. Securing heavy furniture to the wall, installing baby gates at stairways, and keeping hazardous items, such as cleaning supplies and sharp objects, safely stored are all crucial practices. Many parents find it helpful to regularly inspect the home from the baby's level, assessing any new areas they may access as they grow. A safe play area, with soft flooring and age-appropriate toys, provides a space for the baby to explore and develop motor skills within a secure environment.

Maintaining a healthy home environment also involves monitoring and minimizing exposure to harmful substances. Avoiding smoking inside the home and limiting exposure to strong fragrances, aerosols, and harsh chemicals can support respiratory health for both mother and baby. If there are pets in the home, keeping their areas clean and grooming them regularly can reduce the risk of allergen exposure and help maintain hygiene. Many parents also choose to keep indoor shoes separate from outdoor shoes to minimize the dirt and pollutants tracked into the home, which is particularly beneficial for families with babies or young children who spend time on the floor.

Safe and healthy home practices before and after birth encompass a wide range of considerations, from cleanliness and organization to emotional well-being and safety precautions. By prioritizing these practices, families create a home environment that supports both the physical and emotional needs of the mother and baby. As the family adjusts to new routines, maintaining these practices helps establish a stable, nurturing space where each member can feel secure and supported. Creating a healthy home environment ultimately fosters a foundation of wellness and connection, allowing parents to navigate the demands of early parenthood with confidence and resilience.

## The Impact of Sleep on Wellness

The impact of sleep on wellness before and after birth is profound, as sleep plays a crucial role in both physical health and mental well-being. During pregnancy, sleep is essential for the development of the fetus and the health of the mother, influencing hormone regulation, emotional stability, and overall energy levels. After childbirth, sleep remains a critical factor for recovery and for managing the demands of caring for a newborn. The quality and quantity of sleep during these periods directly impact immune function, mood regulation, cognitive abilities, and stress levels, making it one of the most important aspects of prenatal and postpartum wellness.

During pregnancy, sleep is often disrupted by physical discomfort, hormonal changes, and emotional factors such as anxiety and anticipation about the upcoming birth. In the first trimester, hormonal shifts, especially increases in progesterone, lead to increased fatigue and a need for more rest. This hormonal change prepares the body to support fetal growth but can also interfere with the quality of sleep. As pregnancy progresses, the physical changes, such as weight gain, back pain, and frequent urination due to pressure on the bladder, make it difficult for mothers to get uninterrupted rest. For instance, as the abdomen expands, finding a comfortable sleeping position becomes challenging, often leading to increased nighttime awakenings. Sleeping on the side, especially the left side, is typically recommended to improve blood flow to the fetus, uterus, and kidneys, but adjusting to this position can require time and patience.

Sleep during pregnancy also plays a significant role in managing blood pressure, which is crucial for preventing conditions like preeclampsia. Research indicates that insufficient or poor-quality sleep may be associated with increased risks of hypertension, gestational diabetes, and preeclampsia, as disrupted sleep can influence hormone levels that regulate blood pressure. Moreover, quality sleep supports the immune system, helping mothers stay healthier by fighting off common illnesses that could impact pregnancy. A rested body and a balanced immune response reduce the likelihood of infections and support overall fetal development. Therefore, prioritizing adequate sleep during pregnancy contributes not only to immediate well-being but also to a healthier pregnancy journey.

In terms of mental health, sleep is essential for managing the emotional fluctuations that come with pregnancy. Sleep deprivation or poor sleep quality can amplify stress, anxiety, and irritability, affecting emotional resilience and stability. Adequate sleep supports the brain's regulation of stress hormones like cortisol, which helps in coping with day-to-day challenges more effectively. Additionally, the brain processes emotions and solidifies memories during sleep, which is critical for expectant mothers adjusting to the emotional shifts and changes in their lives. Pregnant women who experience consistent, restorative sleep are more likely to maintain a positive outlook and emotional stability, which is beneficial for both maternal well-being and fetal development. Emotional well-being during pregnancy is crucial, as it reduces stress and lowers the likelihood of postpartum depression, making good sleep a valuable aspect of mental health.

After birth, the sleep needs of the mother change considerably due to the physical recovery required and the caregiving demands of a newborn. The postpartum period, also known as the fourth trimester, is marked by intense sleep disruptions for both the mother and the baby. A newborn's sleep schedule, which does not follow a circadian rhythm initially, typically involves frequent waking throughout the day and night, leading to fragmented sleep for the mother. As a result, postpartum sleep deprivation is common and can significantly impact the mother's physical recovery, immune function, and mental health. Sleep deprivation can slow down the body's healing process, particularly for mothers recovering from childbirth or cesarean section. Insufficient sleep can weaken the immune system, making mothers more susceptible to infections and illnesses when they are already vulnerable.

Sleep loss after birth also affects the production of essential hormones, such as oxytocin and prolactin, which support breastfeeding. Oxytocin, the "bonding hormone," is vital for milk ejection and for establishing a strong emotional connection between mother and baby. Prolactin, a hormone released during sleep, promotes milk production, and a lack of sleep can lead to decreased milk supply, adding stress to the breastfeeding process. Additionally, sleep disturbances affect the body's cortisol levels, which can result in increased stress, irritability, and fatigue, making it challenging for mothers to cope with the demands of early motherhood. In this way, sleep is not only critical for physical recovery but also plays a key role in fostering the bond between mother and child, as well as supporting the baby's nutritional needs through breastfeeding.

Mental health in the postpartum period is closely tied to sleep quality, with many studies indicating that poor sleep contributes to higher rates of postpartum depression, anxiety, and mood swings. Sleep deprivation affects neurotransmitter function and disrupts emotional regulation, which increases the risk of experiencing mood-related challenges. A new mother's ability to think, make decisions, and respond to her baby's needs is compromised when she is sleep-deprived. Furthermore, a lack of sleep affects cognitive functions such as memory, concentration, and problem-solving, making it difficult to manage daily tasks and routines. In many cases, postpartum depression is exacerbated by chronic sleep deprivation, which impairs the mother's resilience and ability to cope with stress. Mothers who are well-rested are better able to regulate their emotions, feel more optimistic, and interact with their newborns in a nurturing way, which contributes positively to the baby's development and emotional security.

Sleep for the newborn is equally important, as it is during sleep that much of a baby's growth and brain development occur. Newborns spend more time in rapid eye movement (REM) sleep, a phase of sleep associated with memory consolidation and neural growth. During these periods, babies process sensory experiences, helping them make sense of their environment and forming the basis of early learning. Additionally, sleep helps regulate the release of growth hormones, which are essential for physical development in infants. A well-rested newborn is often calmer, more alert, and better able to engage with their surroundings, supporting social and cognitive growth. Given that a baby's sleep schedule can be unpredictable in the first few months, new parents often need to adjust their routines and find opportunities to rest when the baby is sleeping.

Creating a sleep-friendly environment in the home can help improve sleep quality for both the mother and the baby. For mothers, this means setting up a comfortable, quiet, and dimly lit sleep area that is conducive to rest. Using blackout curtains, minimizing screen time before bed, and incorporating relaxation techniques, such as deep breathing or meditation, can make it easier to fall asleep and achieve more restorative rest. Many parents find it beneficial to sleep in shifts or to share nighttime responsibilities, allowing each parent to get a longer stretch of uninterrupted sleep. Additionally, developing a consistent bedtime routine, such as having a warm bath, practising relaxation techniques, and maintaining a regular sleep schedule, helps the mother's body adjust to a more predictable sleep pattern, even if it is shorter than her usual sleep duration.

For the newborn, safe sleep practices are critical for wellness, as they reduce the risk of sudden infant death syndrome (SIDS). The American

Academy of Pediatrics recommends placing the baby on their back to sleep, using a firm sleep surface, and keeping the crib free of loose bedding or stuffed animals. A consistent sleep routine can also help signal to the baby that it is time for rest, even if they do not yet follow a typical day-night schedule. Some parents find that swaddling or using white noise can help soothe the baby and promote longer sleep periods. As the baby grows, establishing a gentle bedtime routine that includes calming activities like reading or gentle rocking can help create positive sleep associations and make it easier for them to settle into a regular sleep pattern.

In addition to home routines, support from partners, family members, or friends can significantly impact the quality of sleep for new mothers. Sharing caregiving duties, arranging for someone to care for the baby while the mother naps, or seeking help with household responsibilities can alleviate the demands on the mother and allow for more opportunities to rest. Family members and friends can also support mental wellness by providing emotional support, allowing mothers to express concerns or frustrations that may otherwise lead to stress and sleep disturbances. By ensuring that new mothers have support and feel emotionally connected to those around them, they are better able to manage their physical and emotional health, contributing positively to their overall well-being.

Sleep remains a vital component of wellness, impacting physical health, mental resilience, emotional stability, and the capacity to care for a newborn. Before birth, prioritizing sleep enables the mother's body to support fetal growth, regulates essential hormones, and promotes mental clarity and emotional balance. After birth, sleep takes on an even more critical role, as it influences the mother's recovery, hormonal balance, and ability to bond with the baby. Establishing routines, fostering a supportive home environment, and seeking help when needed all contribute to better sleep quality and, in turn, to a healthier and more positive postpartum experience. By understanding the value of sleep and making it a priority, mothers can significantly enhance their well-being and

create a stable foundation for their baby's growth
and development.

# CHAPTER 4: BONDING AND BEYOND

## Preparing for Baby: What You Need to Know

Bringing a new baby into the world is both exciting and overwhelming, and preparation can make a significant difference. Here's a comprehensive list of things to consider as you get ready for your little one's arrival, from creating a safe, comfortable space to planning for the early days of newborn care.

o   **Setting Up a Nursery**

✓   Safe Sleeping Arrangements: Choose a crib or bassinet that meets the latest safety standards. Ensure the mattress is firm and fitted, and avoid loose bedding, pillows, or stuffed animals.

✓   Changing Station: Set up a dedicated area with diapers, wipes, and extra clothes within easy reach. A safe, stable changing table or a changing pad on a dresser works well.

✓ Storage Solutions: Babies require a surprising amount of stuff! Use bins, drawers, and shelves to organize clothing, blankets, toys, and supplies.

✓ Lighting and Noise Control: Consider a soft nightlight and a white noise machine to create a soothing environment for sleep.

o **Essentials for Feeding**

✓ Breastfeeding Supplies: Invest in nursing bras, pads, a breast pump (if needed), and nipple cream to support breastfeeding. Lactation consultants can also offer valuable guidance.

✓ Bottle-Feeding Supplies: Choose bottles that suit your baby's needs. You may need a few different nipples to find one that works best, as well as a bottle brush for easy cleaning.

✓ Formula Options: If you're using formula, consult your paediatrician to choose the best type for your baby. Have a supply on hand for convenience.

✓      Burp Cloths: Babies can be messy eaters. Stock up on burp cloths or bibs to protect your clothes and keep your baby comfortable during feeds.

o      **Clothing and Linens**

✓      Newborn Clothes: Start with essentials like onesies, sleepers, hats, and socks. Choose soft, breathable fabrics that are gentle on newborn skin.

✓      Seasonal Needs: Depending on the weather, consider layering options or bundling clothes to keep your baby comfortable in any season.

✓      Bedding and Blankets: Have fitted crib sheets, swaddle blankets, and a few extra baby blankets for added warmth. Muslin blankets are great for swaddling, while thicker blankets can be used during supervised time.

✓      Laundry Considerations: Newborns can go through several outfits and linens each day. Use a gentle, fragrance-free detergent designed for sensitive skin.


o      **Bathing and Hygiene**

✓      Bathing Supplies: Invest in a baby bathtub or a sink insert for safer bathing. Gather mild, baby-safe soap, a soft washcloth, and a hooded towel.

✓      Diapering Needs: Stock up on diapers (cloth or disposable) in newborn size, but don't buy too many, as babies grow fast. Keep wipes and a diaper cream handy for easy access.

✓      Nail Clippers and Grooming Kit: Baby nails grow quickly and are often sharp. A small nail clipper, soft brush, and nasal aspirator are great to have on hand.

✓      First Aid Supplies: Prepare a baby-specific first aid kit, including a thermometer, gentle saline drops, and any recommended medications for newborns.

o        **Health and Safety Essentials**

✓        Car Seat: A rear-facing infant car seat is essential. Ensure it is properly installed and meets safety regulations.

✓        Baby Monitor: A baby monitor offers peace of mind, whether audio or video, especially if your baby will sleep in a separate room.

✓        Baby-Proofing Supplies: While babies don't crawl right away, begin preparing by installing outlet covers, and corner protectors, and securing heavy furniture to the wall.

✓        Emergency Contacts and Resources: Keep emergency numbers readily accessible, including your paediatrician, poison control, and nearby family or friends who can offer support.

o        **Emotional and Practical Preparation**

✓        Rest and Self-Care: Take time to rest and recharge, especially during the last few weeks. Sleep can be challenging post-birth, so prioritizing self-care is crucial.

✓        Communication with Partner or Support Network: Discuss expectations and create a support plan with your partner, family, or friends to help manage daily tasks after the baby arrives.

✓      Mindfulness and Emotional Health: Pregnancy and early parenthood can bring up a range of emotions. Consider journaling, meditating, or joining a support group to process your feelings.

o      **Newborn Care and Parenting Resources**

✓      Prenatal and Parenting Classes: Many hospitals offer classes on newborn care, breastfeeding, and CPR. Virtual resources are also available for convenience.

✓      Books and Online Resources: Reading up on baby care, sleep strategies, and developmental milestones can help you feel more prepared.

✓      Paediatrician Selection: Choose a paediatrician in advance and schedule a consultation to ensure you're comfortable with their approach to newborn care.

✓ Postpartum Support: Keep information on postpartum care handy, and consider contacting a lactation consultant or mental health counsellor if needed.

o **Financial and Legal Planning**

✓ Budgeting for Baby: Estimate costs for baby supplies, health care, and potential childcare. Creating a budget in advance can ease financial stress.

✓ Insurance and Benefits: Verify health insurance coverage for both you and your baby. Look into any parental leave policies, benefits, or other support options.

✓ Legal Considerations: Draft or update wills, assign a guardian, and consider setting up a savings account for future needs.

o **Preparing Your Home and Routine**

✓ Clean and Organize: Declutter your living spaces to make room for baby gear and supplies.

A clean, organized home will also make the transition smoother.

✓ Meal Preparation: Prepare and freeze meals for the early postpartum days when cooking may be challenging. Quick, nutritious options will be a lifesaver.

✓ Setting up Feeding and Comfort Zones: Create a cosy spot with nursing pillows, blankets, and snacks for those long feeding sessions. Having a designated area for baby care also simplifies routines.

✓ Pet and Sibling Preparation: If you have pets or older children, prepare them for the arrival of the baby by establishing boundaries, schedules, and routines.

o **Flexibility and Adaptability**

✓ Keeping an Open Mind: Every baby is unique, and even the best-laid plans might need adjustments. Being flexible and patient can ease the transition to new parenthood.

✓ Recognizing Support Needs: There's no shame in asking for help, whether it's childcare, housework, or emotional support. Embrace your community as you adjust to this new chapter.

✓ Accepting Change: Parenthood changes daily routines, priorities, and self-identity. Allow yourself to grow with these changes, embracing the journey as you learn and adapt.

Preparing for a baby involves more than just collecting items; it's a holistic process of creating a supportive environment, establishing routines, and readying yourself emotionally and practically. Embrace each step with patience, knowing that flexibility, self-care, and connection with others are key to a smooth transition into parenthood.

## The Importance of Connection Postpartum

The postpartum period is a time of immense joy, change, and vulnerability as new parents adjust to life with their baby. In this delicate phase, connection becomes a crucial foundation for both mental health and overall well-being. Building and nurturing connections with a partner, family, friends, and even with oneself and the baby can help reduce feelings of isolation, promote emotional resilience, and make the transition to parenthood smoother and more fulfilling.

One of the most important connections postpartum is between partners. The shared experience of parenthood can strengthen bonds as each person finds their role in the new family structure. Open communication, sharing responsibilities, and carving out time to check in with each other are all essential in maintaining closeness and support. This mutual connection creates a safe space for both partners to express their needs, feel seen, and find balance amidst the demands of caring for a newborn.

Connecting with family and friends is equally valuable, as they can offer practical help, reassurance, and companionship. Whether it's a friend who drops off a meal, a parent who watches the baby while you take a nap or a call with a loved one to share how you're feeling, these moments help new parents feel supported. Accepting help can be difficult for some, but leaning on others allows for much-needed rest and relief from the demands of constant caregiving.

Joining a community of other new parents, either online or in person, can also be a source of encouragement and understanding. Postpartum groups, breastfeeding circles, or even virtual parenting forums provide a space for sharing experiences, voicing concerns, and gaining advice. This sense of community reminds new parents that they are not alone, helping them feel validated in the challenges and joys they encounter.

Perhaps the most transformative connection is the bond with the baby. Building this bond takes time, patience, and presence, as both parent and baby adjust to each other's rhythms. Moments of skin-to-skin contact, eye contact, and gentle communication help deepen this attachment, creating a foundation of security and trust for the baby and a source of profound love and purpose for the parent.

Finally, connection with oneself is vital. Acknowledging and tending to personal needs, seeking quiet moments for reflection, and embracing self-compassion allow new parents to stay grounded. Self-connection replenishes emotional reserves, helping parents remain resilient and present for their babies and loved ones.

In the postpartum period, connection is a lifeline that nurtures, strengthens, and sustains both parent and child, transforming the experience of early parenthood into one of shared support, joy, and mutual growth.

## Building a Support System

The transition to parenthood is full of excitement, challenges, and unexpected twists. A strong support system can make a world of difference, providing emotional, practical, and informational help when it's most needed. Building this network of support isn't just beneficial—it's essential for parents' well-being and resilience, as well as for nurturing a thriving family environment. Below are some key considerations and strategies for creating a reliable and uplifting support system.

- ○ **Identify Your Support Needs**

- ✓ Emotional Support: Having people you can talk to about the joys and stresses of parenthood is invaluable. Friends, family members, or support groups that provide non-judgmental listening, empathy, and encouragement help reduce isolation and boost confidence.
- ✓ Practical Support: From running errands to helping with household chores, practical support lightens the load and allows parents to focus on bonding with their baby. Practical support can come from neighbours, friends, family, or even hired help like postpartum doulas.
- ✓ Informational Support: Parenting is full of questions, especially in the early days. Access to credible information, whether through experienced parents, lactation consultants, or paediatricians, can provide reassurance and guidance for the many unknowns.

**Build a Circle of Trusted People**

✓ Family and Friends: Family members and close friends are often the first people parents turn to for support. While they may not all live nearby, having a few people you can count on for a quick chat, advice, or assistance makes a big difference. Let loved ones know about your specific needs, whether it's babysitting, meal help, or just being a listening ear.

✓ Parenting Peers: Joining a group of other new parents offers shared understanding and camaraderie. Whether it's an online community, a local mommy-and-me class, or a postpartum group, having a space where people "get it" can be incredibly comforting.

✓ Professional Support: Consider professionals like lactation consultants, postpartum doulas, or mental health counsellors as valuable members of your support system. These individuals provide specialized care, advice, and coping tools. For ongoing concerns or mental health challenges, a counsellor or therapist can offer tailored support and stress-relief techniques.

o **Establish Open Communication**

✓ Express Your Needs Clearly: People can't help unless they know what you need. Be clear and honest about what would make a difference, whether it's babysitting, meals, or just a phone call to check-in. Letting others know your boundaries and needs can reduce frustration and enhance understanding.

✓ Set Boundaries: While support is important, it's equally vital to protect your family's space and time. Don't hesitate to set limits if someone's involvement becomes overwhelming or if certain support doesn't feel beneficial.

✓ Be Open to Feedback: Sometimes, well-meaning advice may feel overwhelming or unsolicited. Try to stay open to feedback but also be discerning, taking what resonates and setting aside what doesn't fit your family's needs or values.

o **Cultivate Community Connections**

✓ Local Parent Groups and Classes: Many communities offer classes or groups that allow new parents to meet others nearby. These gatherings are a great way to build local connections, exchange advice, and set up playdates.

- ✓ Online Communities: Social media and parenting forums can be a lifeline, especially for those in rural or isolated areas. From breastfeeding groups to sleep support, online communities offer a wealth of resources, real-time feedback, and shared experiences.

- ✓ Childcare Networks: For parents returning to work, having trusted childcare arrangements is crucial. Look for support among family members, neighbours, or daycare centres and research thoroughly to find a fit that aligns with your family's needs and values.

- ○ **Take Advantage of Resources and Services**

- ✓ Health and Wellness Services: Local health clinics or pediatric offices often provide support services like lactation consultations, parenting classes, and postpartum check-ins. Many hospitals also offer new parent support groups, which are a good way to access resources and meet other parents.

✓ Meal Delivery and Household Help: Consider meal-prep services, grocery delivery, or even hiring a house cleaner periodically. Services like these give you more time to focus on bonding with your baby and ensure you're not overwhelmed by daily tasks.

✓ Mental Health Resources: Postpartum emotions can be intense, and professional help can provide essential support. Mental health providers, support hotlines, and postpartum specialists are invaluable resources for navigating difficult feelings or anxiety.

o **Build Self-Support and Personal Boundaries**

✓ Self-Care Practices: A support system isn't only about others; it's also about developing ways to care for yourself. Prioritize sleep, eat nourishing foods, and set aside small moments for activities you enjoy, whether it's reading a book, journaling, or going for a walk.

✓ Personal Boundaries: Be mindful of your energy and time. Setting boundaries with others helps you preserve energy for yourself and your family, creating a balanced support system that doesn't drain you.

✓ Reach Out When Needed: Sometimes asking for help can be difficult, but it's important to remember that it's okay to lean on others. Allowing yourself to ask for support is not a weakness—it's a strength that acknowledges the importance of shared care and community.

o **Encourage Mutual Support**

✓ Reciprocal Relationships: A support system functions best when relationships are mutual. Offering help to friends and family when they need it builds a foundation of trust and reciprocity. Small gestures, like checking in or offering a hand, contribute to a strong, sustainable network.

✓ Celebrate Wins Together: Sharing milestones, baby's firsts, or even small parenting successes strengthens bonds and makes others feel part of your journey. Celebrating the good moments can foster joy and positivity in your support circle.

✓ Cultivate Gratitude: Expressing thanks to those who support you fosters warmth and appreciation in your relationships. Whether it's a thank-you note, a phone call, or an invite to coffee, letting people know they're appreciated strengthens connections and keeps them vibrant.

o **Stay Adaptable and Open**

✓ Reevaluate as Needed: As your baby grows, your support needs may change. Keep communication open with your support system, adjusting your needs or boundaries as circumstances shift.

✓ Embrace Change: Life with a new baby often requires flexibility. Stay open to unexpected support from surprising sources, and remember that it's okay to adjust your support circle over time.

✓ Trust the Process: Building a solid support system takes time and effort, but it's a worthwhile investment. Nurture these connections, trusting that they will create a stable foundation of love and resilience for you and your family.

Building a support system is not just about finding people to lean on but about creating a nurturing network that uplifts, empowers, and sustains you as a parent. By combining family, friends, community resources, and self-care practices, you can build a network of care that helps you navigate the challenges of parenthood while celebrating its countless joys. With a well-rounded support system in place, you're better equipped to meet the needs of both yourself and your child, fostering a positive environment for everyone in the family to thrive.

## Early development: caring for your baby's health

The first months of a baby's life are critical for growth and development, as their bodies and minds rapidly adapt to the world around them. Caring for a baby's health in this early stage requires attention to physical needs, emotional nurturing, and consistent wellness routines that help lay a foundation for lifelong well-being. Below are key areas to consider when supporting a baby's early development.

## Nutrition and Feeding

Newborns depend on breast milk or formula for all their nutritional needs. Breast milk provides antibodies that boost a baby's immune system, while formula offers a nutritious alternative if breastfeeding isn't possible or preferred. Feeding on demand, typically every 2-3 hours, ensures babies get the nutrients they need to grow and thrive. Paying attention to your baby's hunger cues, like rooting or sucking motions, and working with a paediatrician for guidance can help you establish a feeding routine that supports optimal growth.

## Sleep and Routine

Sleep is essential for newborns, with babies needing about 16-18 hours of sleep per day. Creating a calm, dark, and quiet sleep environment aids restful sleep and encourages a natural sleep rhythm. Babies are safest sleeping on their backs on a firm mattress, with no loose bedding or toys, to reduce the risk of Sudden Infant Death Syndrome (SIDS). Over time, a gentle bedtime routine—like a bath, story, or lullaby—can help your baby recognize when it's time to wind down.

## Health Checkups and Immunizations

Regular checkups are crucial in monitoring a baby's health, growth, and developmental milestones. During these visits, paediatricians track weight, length, and head circumference and answer any questions you may have. Immunizations also play a vital role in protecting babies from serious diseases; these are typically administered in the first few months and follow a recommended schedule. Staying informed about your baby's health milestones and vaccination appointments will help you stay proactive in supporting their well-being.

## Bonding and Emotional Health

Early interactions between you and your baby promote emotional health and cognitive development. Skin-to-skin contact, soothing sounds, eye contact, and gentle touch build trust and create a secure bond, laying a foundation for emotional resilience. Babies respond to the warmth and security provided by caregivers, which enhances brain development and social skills over time.

## Physical Development and Tummy Time

Physical development is important for muscle strength and coordination. Supervised tummy time encourages motor skills as babies learn to lift their heads, strengthening their neck and shoulder muscles. Initially, a few minutes a day is enough, gradually increasing as your baby becomes more comfortable. Additionally, talking, singing, and playing with your baby stimulate their senses and create moments of connection that support overall development.

Caring for your baby's health is about creating a safe, nurturing, and supportive environment where they can grow, explore, and feel secure. By focusing on nutrition, sleep, health checkups, bonding, and physical activity, you'll be giving your baby a strong foundation for a happy, healthy future.

# CONCLUSION

## Embracing the Journey Together

As you come to the end of *The Well Mom, Well Baby Guide: Simple, Effective Strategies for a Happy Journey Together*, know that you have gained practical tools, gentle insights, and a wealth of support for the journey ahead. The adventure of parenthood is filled with joy, growth, and unique challenges. From birth through the first tender years, the relationship you build with your baby is a cornerstone of their development and well-being, and equally important is how you care for yourself. This journey isn't just about thriving as a parent but also about flourishing as an individual. This conclusion aims to reaffirm that commitment to wellness for both mom and baby, and to remind you that small, consistent actions can make all the difference.

## Reaffirming the Foundation of Connection and Care

Each stage of your child's development comes with moments of excitement, growth, and change. But just as importantly, it comes with the need for connection and care. The bonds formed between you and your baby don't simply happen—they are nurtured through daily routines, loving interactions, and shared moments. Whether it's in feeding, bedtime rituals, play, or moments of quiet bonding, these actions communicate safety, love, and trust, fostering a secure attachment that will support your baby's emotional health for years to come. And remember, the love and care you give to yourself is as vital as what you give to your child. Self-care is not a luxury; it's an essential practice that strengthens you and makes you a better, happier parent.

## Nurturing Flexibility and Growth

Parenthood is often described as one of life's greatest teachers, bringing lessons in patience, flexibility, and resilience. Along the way, it's natural to feel a mix of emotions—joy, doubt, pride, and even uncertainty. There is no one right way to approach each challenge, and even with the best of plans, situations will arise that require adaptability. Embrace each moment as an opportunity to learn and grow, knowing that your intuition and compassion will guide you. By practising flexibility, you allow yourself to adjust and embrace changes, creating a healthy environment for your family to grow together.

## Building a strong, supportive network

In parenting, as in life, community plays a powerful role. A support system offers practical help, emotional support, and a sense of belonging. As your child grows, your network will be there to share milestones, offer advice, and support you through life's ups and downs. Remember, you're not alone on this journey. Relying on friends, family, and even professional guidance is a strength, not a weakness. Each relationship you nurture becomes part of the larger network that will uplift you and your family, creating a foundation of love and encouragement.

## Embracing the adventure ahead

While every parenting journey is unique, the moments of shared laughter, new discoveries, and quiet connection define the beauty of family life. Let this guide serve as a gentle reminder that it's okay to move at your own pace, celebrate the small victories, and find joy in each phase. The journey you're on is one of profound growth—for you, your baby, and your entire family.

As you close this book, take a moment to feel proud of the commitment you're making to your child and yourself. Parenthood is a continuous path of learning and transformation, with each day bringing new challenges, surprises, and joys. Trust in yourself, lean into your support system, and enjoy the journey as you and your child grow and thrive together. The well-being of both mom and baby is a journey that doesn't end here—it's a path of ongoing love, care, and shared happiness that will continue to blossom with every new stage and experience.